HEALING TRADITIONS
Ancestral Echoes For Wise Living Today.

*

By Silvia Atim

Healing Traditions: Ancestral Echoes For Wise Living Today.

Copyright © <2024> <Silvia Atim>

All rights reserved. No part of this book may be reproduced, scanned, or distributed in any printed or electronic form without permission. Please do not participate in or encourage piracy of copyrighted materials in violation of the author's rights. Some names, places, characters and incidents may be fictitious.

Dedicated to all those searching for inner peace

Foreword

Healing Traditions: Ancestral Echoes for Wise Living Today.

In Africa, words hold great significance. They can be chanted as blessings or curses, used for caution or guidance. Proverbs, known as "caro lok" in my Acholi tribe, are words of wisdom spoken by our ancestors, passed down through generations to serve as valuable tools for education and guidance in our daily lives.

Introduction

In the gentle glow of the *wang oo* (campfire), as shadows flickered and the comforting scent of roasted maize and cassava filled the air, we gathered under the evening sky. The elders shared stories, gems of wisdom drawn from their experience and tradition. These gatherings were more than mere entertainment; they were our guiding stars, teaching us strength, kindness, and resilience. The elders would tell stories filled with meaning, often after moments of discipline or advice, explaining the importance of certain behaviors and how to live with integrity, compassion, and wisdom.

Living in America today, I find these stories to be as profoundly relevant as ever. This book brings together those life-shaping tales, interwoven with reflections on how their timeless messages help me navigate today's challenges. From confronting low self-esteem, shame, and humility to overcoming anxiety, anger, and doubt, these stories provide valuable tools for managing the stresses of modern life. Each story serves as a bridge between the wisdom of the past and the complexities of contemporary American life—reminding us that while times may change, the principles of a meaningful life remain constant.

Proverb 1

"You don't insult the mouth of the crocodile while you're still crossing the river."-An African Proverb.

This proverb teaches the importance of caution, respect, and awareness in difficult or dangerous situations. It advises against provoking or offending those who have power over you, especially when you are still dependent on them or in a vulnerable position.

A personal story

When I first moved to America and started a new job, everything felt overwhelming. The workplace culture was so different from what I was used to, and despite my best efforts, I felt isolated. My colleagues seemed to have an unspoken understanding of things that I couldn't quite grasp. There were times when I misunderstood what was expected of me, and I found myself feeling overlooked or even bullied by some of my coworkers, who seemed to ignore me or treat me like an outsider.

I started to question if I had made the right choice. The feeling of not belonging grew stronger, and at times, I seriously considered leaving the job. But one evening, as I sat quietly reflecting on everything, I remembered the story my grandfather once told me: *"You don't insult the mouth of the crocodile while you're still crossing the river."* I realized that I was still in the "river," new to the job and to the culture, and I needed to exercise patience instead of rushing to make a decision out of frustration.

Instead of giving up, I decided to take a step back. I focused on learning more about the workplace dynamics, observing how others navigated the challenges I was facing, and asking for guidance when I needed it. Slowly, I began to understand the way things worked and how to communicate better with my colleagues. The bullying and misunderstandings lessened as I showed more patience and resilience, giving myself time to grow into the role rather than making a hasty exit.

That period of doubt and frustration taught me a valuable lesson in exercising patience. Like the crocodile in my grandfather's story, I learned that it's wise to wait and learn when you're still crossing unfamiliar territory. With time, things improved, and I found my place in the job, no longer feeling the urge to leave but instead feeling stronger and more confident.

Lessons it teaches:
1. **Caution in Difficult Situations**: When you're facing a challenge or are in a vulnerable position, it's wise not to create more trouble by angering or disrespecting those who hold power, influence, or control in that situation.
2. **Respect for Authority**: This proverb encourages showing respect for authority or people in positions of power, particularly when you still need their assistance or are relying on them for your safety or success.
3. **Patience and Strategy**: Sometimes, it's better to wait for the right time to act or voice your opinions. While

crossing the river, it's best to remain focused on the task at hand rather than engaging in risky behavior that could jeopardize your safety.
4. **Timing and Discernment**: The proverb teaches that timing is key. It's important to choose when and how to address conflict, and some situations require discretion and careful planning to avoid negative consequences.

In essence, this proverb reminds us to be mindful of our actions and words, especially when we are still navigating challenging or risky situations.

Reflection Questions:
1. The proverb, "You don't insult the mouth of the crocodile while you're still crossing the river," emphasizes the importance of patience and caution in difficult situations. How do you interpret this proverb, and can you think of a situation where acting impulsively could have made things worse?
2. In what ways do you think this proverb applies to professional or personal relationships, especially when dealing with authority figures or people who have influence over your situation? How can patience be a strength in these circumstances?
3. Have you ever experienced a situation where you felt mistreated or misunderstood, and how did you balance your desire to react with the wisdom of waiting for the right moment to address the issue? How might this proverb guide someone in a similar situation?
4. The proverb "You don't insult the mouth of the crocodile while you're still crossing the river" teaches the value of timing and caution. How do you assess when it is the right moment to speak up in a tense or

risky situation? What strategies can you use to ensure your actions or words are measured and thoughtful?
5. Sometimes, patience requires restraint even when we feel we are in the right. Can you think of a time when holding back your words or actions allowed you to avoid unnecessary conflict or gain a more favorable outcome? How did waiting help you navigate the situation better?

Proverb 2

"An elephant never fails to carry its tusk.'-An African proverb."

Embracing Responsibilities:

Today, we will explore the African proverb, "An elephant never fails to carry its tusks." This saying reminds us that, like elephants who proudly bear their tusks, we each have responsibilities that we must embrace. The tusks represent the burdens we carry, but they also symbolize our strength and commitment to fulfilling our roles within our families and communities.

A Personal Story

In my village in Madi Opei, chores were a shared responsibility within the family. Fetching water, gathering firewood, and preparing meals for the day were tasks we all took on. My siblings and I often argued over these duties, especially when it was time to fetch water from the borehole. Each trip involved carrying heavy jerrycans or buckets, and the journey back home could stretch for miles. The task seemed daunting, and at times, the weight of our responsibilities felt overwhelming. But on evenings like these, as we sat by the fireplace, my grandfather, who had overheard our squabbles, would calm us with his gentle words and teach us about responsibility. He would tell us the story of the elephant and its tusks, explaining how the elephant used its tusks for the greater good of the community. Through these lessons, we learned to find purpose in our burdens, understanding that by shouldering our responsibilities, we contributed to the well-being of our family and society.

When I was 28, I unexpectedly became a single mother. Suddenly, I was solely responsible for taking care of my daughter. Many times, I found myself feeling overwhelmed, especially as bills piled up, and self-pity crept in. But despite these challenges, I accepted my responsibility and understood that it was my duty to provide for my child. In today's world, we all have tasks and roles that can sometimes feel burdensome. Whether as a parent, child, teacher, or in any other role, our responsibilities may seem heavy at times. However, it's important to remember that we all contribute to the well-being of our families and society. Just like the elephant's tusks may appear cumbersome but ultimately serve the greater good of the village, we all carry burdens that contribute to the greater good. Whatever your "tusk" may be, may you use it to help those around you and accomplish what is needed.

Lessons it teaches:
1. **The Burden of Responsibility**: In life, we all carry responsibilities that can feel overwhelming, much like the heavy jerrycans we had to carry as children. Sometimes, tasks seem daunting, and we may wish to avoid them, but it's important to recognize that these responsibilities are part of our role in the family and society.
2. **The Value of Perseverance**: Despite the challenges, we always found ways to manage, whether by sharing stories, singing, or taking breaks along the

way. Life may present us with difficult tasks, but we can find comfort and strength in how we approach them—sometimes, it's the small moments of joy that help us endure.
3. **Supporting One Another:** Though we bickered over who should go fetch water, it wasn't because we didn't care, but because the burden felt heavy. This reminds us that it's okay to ask for help or to share the load with others. When we support one another, the challenges become easier to bear.
4. **Each of Us Has a Role:** Just as every member of the family has a role to play, whether it's the father, mother, child, or teacher, we all contribute to the greater good. Our individual tasks may seem burdensome, but they are important in the bigger picture. Like the elephant carrying its tusks, our efforts—however heavy they may seem—serve a greater purpose.
5. **Embracing Our Responsibilities:** Just as the elephant carries its tusks for the good of the village, we must embrace our responsibilities, knowing that they contribute to the well-being of our families and communities. The weight of the tasks we carry may seem heavy at times, but they are part of what helps the world function and improve.

Through these lessons, we can learn to approach life's challenges with resilience, support, and a sense of purpose.

Reflection Questions:
1. An elephant never fails to carry its tusk" emphasizes the idea of accepting and bearing one's responsibilities with strength and dignity. How does this proverb resonate with you, and can you think of a time when you had to carry a heavy responsibility that felt overwhelming? What helped you persevere?

2. What does this proverb teach us about the importance of staying committed to our duties, even when they are difficult or burdensome? How might this mindset be helpful in facing challenges at work, in family life, or in pursuing long-term goals?
3. How do you think this proverb applies to the balance between personal burdens and contributing to the greater good of a community or family? Have you ever experienced a moment when fulfilling your obligations had a positive impact on those around you?
4. "An elephant never fails to carry its tusk" highlights the idea of enduring through life's challenges with perseverance. How do you view the role of patience in carrying out your responsibilities? Can you recall a situation where patience helped you maintain focus and move through a challenging task or phase in your life?
5. The elephant's tusks are integral to its identity, just as our responsibilities often shape who we are. How does the weight of your own responsibilities contribute to your sense of purpose and personal growth? Have there been times when taking on a responsibility, despite its difficulty, led to unexpected growth or learning?

Proverb 3

"Do not attempt what you cannot bring to a good end." -An African Proverb.

This proverb emphasizes the importance of careful planning and understanding one's own abilities and limits. It teaches that before starting any endeavor, one should consider whether they have the resources, knowledge, and determination to complete it successfully. The message encourages thoughtful decision-making, responsibility, and the wisdom of knowing when to proceed and when to step back to avoid failure or unintended consequences.

In essence, it serves as a reminder to set realistic goals and approach tasks with commitment and preparation.

A personal story

When I was young, I had an unforgettable encounter that taught me the importance of understanding the consequences of my actions. One afternoon, while exploring the fields near our village, I stumbled upon a large beehive hanging from a tree. The thought of sweet honey was irresistible, and without fully understanding the risks, I picked up a stick and approached the hive, determined to extract honey on my own.

In my excitement, I didn't consider the danger I was putting myself in. As soon as I disturbed the hive, a swarm of bees emerged, angry and ready to defend their home. I ran as fast as I could, but not before being stung multiple times. The pain was intense, and the experience left me humbled and shaken.

That evening, as I nursed my stings, my grandfather sat me down by the fireplace. With a gentle but wise tone, he shared the proverb, "Do not attempt what you cannot bring to a good end." He told me stories about how every action has consequences, and he emphasized the importance of thinking ahead before diving into something that could bring more harm than good.

Reflecting on this moment, the wisdom of the proverb became clear. Just as I had rushed into something without considering the full consequences, people often make hasty decisions only to find themselves overwhelmed by the pain and challenges that follow. My grandfather's story became a lasting reminder to be thoughtful and intentional, understanding that not every tempting opportunity is worth the risk.

Lessons it teaches:
1. **Importance of Preparation and Realism**: The proverb underscores the necessity of being well-prepared and setting realistic goals. In a fast-paced society like America, where ambition and innovation are celebrated, this lesson encourages individuals to assess their abilities and resources before pursuing major endeavors. It highlights the importance of strategic planning to ensure success rather than diving into projects impulsively.
2. **Commitment and Responsibility**: This saying emphasizes the value of commitment and seeing

things through to completion. In the workplace or personal endeavors, it is crucial to understand the responsibilities involved and make sure one is willing and able to fulfill them. This principle applies to both business ventures and personal commitments, stressing the importance of honoring one's word and following through on promises.

3. **Risk Management and Decision-Making**: The proverb reminds us to weigh the risks and potential outcomes of our actions. In America's environment of entrepreneurial spirit and high-stakes decisions, understanding the limits of one's capabilities helps in making wise, calculated choices. It encourages people to be mindful of the consequences and to avoid overextending themselves to prevent failure or harm.

4. **Resource Management**: Whether it's time, energy, or finances, the proverb advises using resources efficiently and not overcommitting. In a world where burnout is increasingly common, especially in professional settings, understanding how to allocate resources wisely can lead to more sustainable and balanced living.

5. **Ethical and Moral Considerations**: Finally, the lesson speaks to ethical integrity, advising people not to start something they cannot ethically or morally complete. For instance, in leadership or social justice movements, the proverb encourages thoughtfulness and a commitment to achieving positive outcomes rather than initiating actions that could be harmful or unsustainable.

These lessons resonate with modern American values of hard work, responsibility, and ethical leadership, providing guidance on navigating both personal and professional spheres with foresight and accountability.

Reflection Questions:
1. Think about a time when you made a decision without fully considering the potential consequences. How did the outcome shape your understanding of the importance of thinking ahead before taking action?
2. In what areas of your life do you sometimes rush into decisions for immediate gratification, without considering if you can see it through to a successful or safe conclusion? How can you apply the lesson from this proverb to approach those situations more thoughtfully?
3. How does the proverb "Do not attempt what you cannot bring to a good end" relate to personal responsibility, especially when facing tempting but risky choices? How can you remind yourself to pause and reflect before taking action?
4. Reflecting on past decisions, have you ever been in a situation where you wished you had taken more time to weigh the pros and cons? How might that experience influence how you approach decision-making in the future, particularly in situations where the stakes are high?
5. When considering new opportunities or challenges, how do you assess whether you have the resources, time, and commitment to follow through? How can you ensure that your decisions align with your long-term goals and values, rather than being driven by short-term impulses?

Proverb 4

"The sound of the drum depends on the drummer."-An African Proverb.

This African proverb highlights the idea that the outcome of any situation, or the way something is experienced, depends on the person who is responsible for it or in charge of it. Just as a drum's sound is shaped by the skill and influence of the drummer, the results of a task or a situation depend on the choices, actions, and perspective of the individual involved.

This proverb emphasizes personal responsibility and the power of individual influence. It suggests that one's actions, decisions, and approach will ultimately determine the outcome or the way things unfold. It serves as a reminder that we are all in control of our own actions and how we shape the world around us.

A personal story

In my journey as a counselor, I started out learning from many accomplished professionals with years of experience. I was eager to observe their techniques and styles, absorbing as much knowledge as possible. Yet, as I developed in my career, I came to understand that while it was crucial to learn from others, it was equally important to establish my own identity.

I aspired to be authentic in my practice—not merely imitating the approaches of my mentors but merging their teachings with my story, history, personality, and unique voice. I realized that being true to myself would boost my confidence and foster deeper therapeutic connections with my clients. Authenticity in my practice allowed me to deliver messages that were not only meaningful but also genuine and impactful.

The proverb, "The sound of the drum depends on the drummer," became a guiding principle for me. Like a drummer who shapes the rhythm, I recognized that my effectiveness as a counselor was influenced by how I expressed myself and approached my work. I needed to be more than a reflection of others' practices; I had to embrace continuous growth while staying true to my unique style. This authenticity not only helped me connect deeply with clients but also made me feel fulfilled, knowing I was being my true self rather than a copy of someone else's approach.

Lessons it teaches:
1. **Personal Responsibility and Influence**: The outcome of any situation or task depends on the individual who is responsible for it. Just like a drummer controls the sound of the drum, we have the power to shape our own actions and decisions. This teaches us that we are responsible for how we navigate life and the impact we make.
2. **Authenticity and Self-expression**: The proverb emphasizes the importance of being true to yourself. Just as a drummer brings their own unique rhythm, we must embrace our individuality and express our true selves. Trying to imitate others will never create the same impact as being authentic to who we are.

3. **Confidence in Our Abilities**: The sound of the drum is determined by how the drummer plays it, highlighting the need to have confidence in our own abilities. Trusting in our skills and experience allows us to have a positive influence on the situations and people around us.
4. **Shaping Our Own Journey**: Whether it's a career, personal goals, or relationships, we are the ones who shape our path. Just as a drummer can create different rhythms, we can determine the direction and impact of our journey by owning our choices and actions.
5. **Adaptability**: Drummers adjust their playing to match the rhythm and mood of the moment, which reminds us to be adaptable. Life requires flexibility, and our ability to adjust and navigate through different situations is key to success.

These lessons encourage us to be mindful of how we engage with the world and highlight the importance of our individual contribution to every situation.

Reflection Questions

1. How do you take responsibility for the outcomes in your life? In what ways have you shaped your personal or professional journey through your own actions and decisions?
2. When have you tried to imitate someone else's style or approach, and how did it affect your authenticity? How can you embrace your unique qualities to create your own rhythm in life?
3. Think about a time when you felt unsure or lacked confidence. How did that impact the way you handled a situation? What steps can you take to trust in your own abilities and shape your path with more confidence?

4. How do you balance taking responsibility for your actions while also recognizing the influence of external factors or other people in shaping your outcomes? How can you ensure you don't place blame on others while still acknowledging the role of circumstances?
5. Can you think of a time when you embraced your authentic self, even when it was difficult or different from the expectations of others? How did that experience contribute to your growth, and how can you continue to honor your true self moving forward?

Proverb 5

"Glory does not come by calling."-An African Proverb.

Growing up in my village, Madi Opei, within the Acholi tribe, the elders were revered figures who held a central place in our community. They were seen as guardians of tradition, called upon to settle disputes with their words of wisdom. Respect for elders was deeply ingrained in our culture, and any transgression against them was often met with stern consequences.

However, there was one elder, Mzee Okuru, whose life told a different story. I don't recall how he got his nickname, but he was infamous for being perpetually drunk. We would often encounter him staggering along the path after school, singing incoherently or passed out under a tree. As children, we found his antics amusing and would sometimes mischievously throw pebbles his way or try to wake him up, finding joy in our childish games. Despite our disrespectful behavior toward Mzee Okuru, we were never severely reprimanded for treating him in a way that would have been unthinkable for any other elder.

One evening by the *Wang oo* (campfire), my grandfather shared a lesson that resonated with me. He spoke about the importance of self-respect and the effort required to earn the respect of others. "Glory does not come by calling," he said. It became clear that Mzee Okuru, despite his status as an elder, had not earned the reverence typically afforded to people of his age in our village. His actions had diminished the respect he might have commanded, highlighting the truth that genuine honor must be earned through consistent behavior, integrity, and dignity.

This lesson has stayed with me and guided me in my own life journey. It reminds me that to be respected or admired, one must live with intention, build credibility through actions, and continuously strive to uphold the values one wishes to be recognized for. Glory, indeed, does not come by simply demanding it; it is cultivated through how we carry ourselves and treat others.

Lessons it teaches:
1. **Earning Respect Through Action**: In today's fast-paced society, respect and recognition are not given freely based on titles or superficial claims. Instead, they are earned through demonstrated competence, integrity, and consistent hard work. Whether in a professional setting or personal relationships, people gain genuine respect by proving their worth through their deeds rather than merely demanding acknowledgment.
2. **The Value of Perseverance**: This proverb emphasizes the importance of effort and dedication. In an era where instant gratification is often sought, it serves as a reminder that lasting success and glory require sustained commitment. For instance, building a reputable brand or career involves perseverance, learning from failures, and continually striving to improve.
3. **Authenticity and Self-Respect**: To command respect from others, one must first exhibit self-respect and

authenticity. In leadership, for example, true influence comes not from a position of authority but from earning the trust and admiration of others through honest and respectful behavior. This ties into the idea that leaders must set an example and inspire confidence rather than expecting loyalty without demonstrating value.

4. **Humility and Continuous Learning**: The proverb also teaches that seeking glory or recognition without putting in the necessary effort is a futile endeavor. In a modern context, it suggests the importance of humility and the willingness to continually learn and grow. Whether pursuing academic achievements, entrepreneurial success, or personal development, the journey requires dedication and ongoing self-improvement.

Ultimately, this proverb is a call to focus on meaningful contributions and the integrity of one's actions, emphasizing that recognition and honor are natural outcomes of living and working with purpose, commitment, and respect for oneself and others

Reflection Questions
1. Think about a leader or parent you admire. What actions did they take that influenced you, and how can you apply those same principles to your own life?
2. In what areas of your life do you think your actions could better align with the values you promote? What changes can you make today to become a better role model?
3. When have you experienced a moment when talking about your goals wasn't enough to achieve them? How did you shift your focus to action, and what did

you learn from that experience?
4. What steps can you take today to ensure that your actions align with your words? In what areas of your life could you focus more on demonstrating your commitment?
5. Think about a person you admire. How did they earn your respect? What actions did they take to prove their worth, and how can you apply similar principles to your own journey?

Proverb 6

"The beginning is the most important part of the work."-An African Proverb.

This African proverb emphasizes the significance of starting strong. It means that how you begin often sets the tone for the rest of your journey. A well-thought-out and determined start builds a foundation for success, while a careless or hesitant start may make progress difficult. This proverb serves as a reminder that the initial phase of any task or endeavor deserves special attention and effort, as it greatly influences the outcome.

Personal Story

When I was growing up in my village of Madi Opei, we used to study under a large tree. We didn't have books or pens; instead, we wrote numbers on the ground with sticks. When it rained, we would quickly run home to escape the downpour. Our teacher, a middle-aged man, was the only one in the village who spoke English. He wore shorts and a tie, and he would tell us that he had been taught by the British. He would share stories of his time in a "white man's land," and we would listen in awe as he described people with skin the color of ashes, and we longed to see such people ourselves. We called him "Teacher Sir" because that's how he instructed us to address him.

For years, our village struggled with illiteracy, but Teacher Sir believed that education was the key to breaking the cycle of poverty. I remember how, as we continued learning, Teacher Sir was gathering resources to build a proper classroom for us. As the school slowly began to take shape, more villagers noticed the change. They saw Kofi's dedication and the strong foundation he was laying. Over time, the project gained more support, and eventually, our school was completed. It became a hub of learning, transforming the future of our community.

Teacher Sir's commitment to starting strong, with careful planning and focus, ensured the school's lasting success. The proverb, "The beginning is the most important part of the work," was evident throughout the project. Without a solid start, the school would not have stood the test of time or made the lasting impact it did on our community.

Lessons it teaches:
1. **Intentionality Matters**: Start your journey with clear intentions and a focus on your values. When your beginning is strong, it becomes easier to navigate obstacles and stay motivated.
2. **Preparation Sets the Foundation**: The initial investment in preparation and planning often leads to better outcomes. Whether you're starting a career, relationship, or project, investing time and energy at the beginning can prevent many issues down the line.
3. **Overcoming Hesitation**: Sometimes, the fear of starting can paralyze you. This proverb reminds us that beginning is crucial, and we must push past that initial hesitation to create momentum.
4. **Stay Connected to Your Purpose**: A strong beginning, grounded in purpose, keeps you anchored

during times of doubt. It gives you something to look back on and reminds you of why you started in the first place.

This proverb encourages us to invest our best energy and intentions in the first steps of our journey, knowing that this strong foundation can lead to greater achievements. What are your thoughts on this, or have you had a meaningful beginning in your life that shaped your journey?

Reflection Questions

1. Why do you think starting strong can influence the outcome of a project or goal? Can you share a time when a well-planned start made a difference in your success?

2. What strategies can you use to prepare yourself mentally and physically for new challenges or responsibilities?

3. How do you decide what is most important to focus on at the beginning of a new task or journey?

4. What does a successful start look like to you, and how can you measure it?

5. How can you maintain the motivation and energy you have at the start throughout your entire journey?

Proverb 7

"When elephants fight, it is the grass that suffers."-An African Proverb.

The African proverb *"When elephants fight, it is the grass that suffers"* conveys the idea that when powerful people or groups are in conflict, it is the innocent and vulnerable who experience the most harm. Just as the grass is trampled and damaged when large animals battle, those who are not part of the struggle often bear the negative consequences. This proverb emphasizes the importance of recognizing the unintended impact that conflicts between stronger forces can have on bystanders.

Personal Story

Growing up, I had a childhood friend named Adoch. I remember that most mornings, when I woke up, I would find Adoch outside our house eating the leftover food from the night before. My mom would give her the food before heading to the fields at dawn to tend to the garden. Of course, she would also save some food in the pot for us to eat when we woke up hungry. In our village, it was common to save the leftovers from the evening meal for the children to eat in the morning, while the older folks went out early to work in the fields. This would be the food we had until the afternoon when the parents returned and began cooking again for dinner.

I didn't mind Adoch coming to our house nearly every morning, and my mom never hesitated to give her the food. However, one day I overheard my parents talking about Adoch's family. They revealed that Adoch's father was an alcoholic, and he would often drink away the family's food. The couple would fight, and sometimes, Adoch's mother would be badly beaten, leaving her unable to cook. In those times, Adoch's father would eat all the food in the house, leaving nothing for Adoch.

Looking back, I realize that Adoch was a very withdrawn child. She often seemed sick, wore worn-out clothes, and clearly suffered in silence. Now, I can understand that Adoch's difficult home life took a heavy toll on her.

Lessons it teaches:
1. **Recognize the Impact of Conflict**: The proverb serves as a reminder to be mindful of how disputes can hurt innocent bystanders. Whether in families, communities, or even global situations, conflicts often create suffering for those who have no part in them.
2. **Prioritize the Well-being of the Vulnerable**: It's crucial for those in positions of power or authority, like parents in a family, to consider the emotional and physical safety of those who depend on them. Protecting the innocent should always be a priority.
3. **Seek Peaceful Resolutions**: Understanding that conflict can cause widespread damage, this proverb emphasizes the importance of seeking ways to resolve issues peacefully. In family settings, healthy communication and conflict resolution skills can create a more harmonious environment.
4. **Acknowledge and Heal the Wounds**: Those who

suffer as a result of others' conflicts may carry emotional scars. It's essential to acknowledge the hurt, provide support, and find ways to heal and move forward.

This proverb is a powerful reminder of the ripple effects our actions can have on others. It encourages empathy and awareness of the ways our struggles may impact those who are most vulnerable. How do you feel this proverb applies to situations you've witnessed or experienced?

Reflection Questions:

1. Who are the "elephants" and the "grass" in conflicts you've seen or heard about, and how did the conflict impact those who were most vulnerable?

2. What can be done to protect or support the "grass" when powerful individuals or groups are in conflict?

3. Have you ever felt like the "grass" in a difficult situation? How did it affect you, and what support would have made a difference?

4. Why is it important to consider the impact of our actions on those who may be indirectly affected?

5. How can we work toward resolving conflicts in a way that minimizes harm to those who are not directly involved?

Proverb 8

"If you do what you should not do, you will see what you should not see."-An African Proverb.

This African proverb emphasizes that actions have consequences, and engaging in behaviors that are wrong or risky can lead to undesirable or harmful outcomes. It serves as a warning to think carefully before making choices that could bring unintended trouble or distress.

A personal Story

When I was younger, I was often drawn to experiences my elders warned us to avoid. One of their most chilling tales was about the *latal*, or night dancers—witches who ran naked, covered in ashes, performing dark rituals. Our elders insisted we keep our doors locked at night to stay safe, as some villagers even claimed to have been victims of their witchcraft. The stories kept us vigilant, and every evening, we spoke in hushed tones to avoid drawing their attention.

One night, when our parents were away at a neighboring village, I convinced my reluctant friend Adoch to join me in trying to catch a glimpse of a *latal*. Our grandfather, who was watching over us, had gone to bed early, and the moonlight made the night seem less threatening. Quietly, we laid down on our reed mats, waiting for the perfect moment. Feeling brave, we eventually stepped outside, following the distant sound of drums from a celebration. As we walked, curiosity and excitement filled us.

Lost in conversation, we suddenly heard rustling in the bushes ahead. A dark, menacing figure emerged, and panic washed over us. We ran back to our hut, screaming, terrified that we had seen a *latal*. In our village, witnessing one was a bad omen, and I was convinced we had brought misfortune upon ourselves. Reflecting now, I see how curiosity and defiance led us to experiences we were far too young to face.

Lessons it teaches:
1. **The Importance of Boundaries**: The proverb teaches us that there are rules, norms, or ethical boundaries in life for a reason. Overstepping these boundaries can lead to negative consequences or experiences we are not prepared to handle. This can apply to everything from personal relationships to professional behavior, emphasizing the importance of respecting limits.
2. **Mindfulness and Self-Control**: It serves as a reminder to exercise self-discipline and resist temptations that may lead us astray. By being mindful of our actions and making thoughtful choices, we can avoid unnecessary trouble or distress.
3. **Consequences of Risky Behavior**: Engaging in reckless or inappropriate behavior often leads to unintended outcomes, some of which can be life-changing or harmful. This lesson encourages people to think carefully about their decisions and be aware of the possible repercussions.
4. **Avoiding Unnecessary Harm**: The proverb warns that pursuing dangerous or forbidden paths can expose us to situations or knowledge that can be

unsettling or damaging. It promotes the idea of protecting oneself from experiences that may be harmful or burdensome.

Overall, this proverb emphasizes the value of making wise, ethical, and considerate decisions to avoid encountering negative or unforeseen consequences. It reminds us to act responsibly and think about the long-term effects of our actions.

Reflection Questions

1. Have you ever faced a situation where you were tempted to do something you knew was wrong? What guided your decision, and what was the outcome?
2. Why do you think people are often drawn to doing things they know they shouldn't? What can help them make safer choices?
3. How can peer pressure influence our decisions, and what strategies can we use to resist it?
4. What role does listening to the advice of adults or more experienced people play in keeping us safe? Can you think of a time when someone's warning saved you from trouble?
5. What can we learn about the importance of considering consequences before acting on impulses? How might this affect the decisions we make in our daily lives?

Proverb 9

"Wisdom is like a baobab tree; a single person's arms cannot embrace it."-An African Proverb.

This African suggests that wisdom is vast and cannot be fully comprehended or grasped by one person alone. It emphasizes the importance of collective knowledge and the idea that we need to share insights and experiences with others to understand the world more deeply.

Personal Story

Growing up, I was fortunate to have a strong sense of community among my relatives and neighbors. One summer, my cousins and I had a disagreement about the best way to start a garden in our backyard. Each of us had a different idea: some believed that we should plant rows of vegetables and focus on soil quality, while others argued for planting fruit trees and investing in compost.

At first, I was determined to do things my way. I had read a few articles and thought I knew exactly what to do. But as we discussed, our grandmother stepped in and shared stories from her own experiences with gardening in her youth. Then, our neighbor Mr. Johnson, a retired farmer, joined in and talked about his years of cultivating the land. Soon, we found ourselves gathering more people from the neighborhood—each sharing tips, mistakes they had made, and the joys of a bountiful harvest.

We realized that no single person had all the answers. It was the collective wisdom of the group that helped us design a garden that thrived, with a mix of vegetables, fruit trees, and healthy soil practices. That experience taught me that I should never underestimate the power of gathering wisdom from others.

Lessons it teaches:

This proverb highlights that just as a community is needed to support the vast trunk of a baobab tree, gaining true wisdom requires collaboration and the inclusion of diverse perspectives.

1. **Value Collective Knowledge**: Wisdom is vast and multifaceted. We need the perspectives and experiences of others to truly learn and grow.
2. **Be Open to Learning from Others**: Sometimes, we think we know the best way forward, but sharing ideas and listening to others can reveal better paths.
3. **Respect Elders and Communities**: People who have lived through experiences often hold valuable insights. Taking the time to listen to them can teach us more than we ever imagined.

Reflection Questions

1. Why is it important to listen to different perspectives before making a decision? How might this apply to your life right now?
2. How do you think wisdom is shared in your family or community? Are there certain people you turn to for advice, and why?
3. What are the dangers of believing that you have all the answers or refusing to seek advice from others?
4. How can you contribute to the collective wisdom of your community or group, even if you don't think you have much experience?

5. What role does humility play in your ability to learn from others, and how can embracing it improve your decision-making process?

Proverb 10

"A dirty tongue litters its owner."-An African Proverb.

This proverb highlights the impact and consequences of our words. It teaches that using negative, harsh, or hurtful language, as well as spreading falsehoods or gossip, often leads to a damaged reputation and strained relationships for the speaker. This proverb underscores the value of communicating with mindfulness, respect, and honesty, as our words have the power to either elevate or bring disgrace upon us.

A Personal story

In my village in Madi Opei, there was a woman named Min Akech (meaning "mother of Akech"). Everyone knew her for her sharp tongue; she was a master at hurling insults, and people dreaded arguing with her because she could berate you endlessly until you were left speechless. Her verbal attacks and harsh language shocked people, especially in our culture, where using obscenities is frowned upon, particularly when children are within earshot. As a result, people distanced themselves from her, wanting nothing to do with her. She became isolated, as no one wanted to be around her wrath or endure her hurtful words. Her reputation suffered, and even the men avoided her. She remained single and alone until she seemed to realize that using vulgar language doesn't make someone heroic or invincible; rather, it taints one's image. Over time, she started to tone down her behavior.

When I later moved to America, I noticed that vulgar language and obscenities were more common. People referred to it as cursing or used derogatory language, such as calling women names like "bitch,". Regardless of the form, I observed that in workplaces, such behavior can be damaging. Using offensive language in professional environments tarnishes a person's reputation and can hinder career growth, making it difficult to earn promotions or be highly regarded for opportunities. This proverb serves as a universal reminder that the way we speak can either build bridges or burn them, shaping how others perceive and connect with us

Lessons it teaches:
1. **The Power of Words**: Words have lasting effects. They can uplift and inspire, or they can deeply wound and damage relationships. Being mindful of our language helps us foster positive connections.
2. **Reputation Matters**: Harsh or negative speech can damage our character and reputation. People remember how we make them feel, and consistent hurtful communication can lead to social isolation and lost opportunities.
3. **Mindful Communication**: Practicing thoughtful and respectful speech shows emotional maturity and self-control. It's about being aware of how our words affect others and choosing to speak in a way that adds value.
4. **Self-Respect and Dignity**: By maintaining respectful communication, we uphold our own dignity and self-respect. Speaking well of others and refraining from

gossip or insults reflects a strong sense of character.
5. **Conflict Resolution**: When faced with disagreements, choosing calm and constructive words can prevent escalation. It shows wisdom and a commitment to resolving conflicts peacefully rather than fueling them.

Overall, this proverb teaches that our words are a reflection of our inner values. By communicating with integrity and kindness, we not only protect our own reputation but also contribute to a more respectful and harmonious environment.

Reflection questions

Here are five reflection questions you can pose to a class based on the proverb "a dirty tongue litters its owner":

1. Can you recall a time when someone's words either uplifted you or hurt you deeply? How did it impact your relationship with that person?
2. How do you think your choice of words affects the way others perceive and respond to you, both in personal and professional settings?
3. Have you ever experienced or witnessed a situation where negative or harsh language led to consequences, such as damaged relationships or social isolation? What lessons did you learn from that experience?
4. What strategies can you use to remain mindful and respectful when speaking, especially during moments of anger or frustration?
5. In what ways can this proverb inspire you to reflect on and improve your communication habits in order to strengthen your connections with others?

Proverb 11

"The strength of a fish is in the water."-An African Proverb.

This proverb emphasizes the importance of being in an environment that supports one's abilities and potential. Just as a fish is strong and capable when in water but becomes vulnerable and powerless when taken out of it, people thrive when they are in circumstances or places that nurture their talents and strengths. The proverb highlights the significance of being mindful of where we place ourselves and how our surroundings impact our well-being and success.

A Personal story

Growing up in my village of Madi Opei, I remember a childhood friend named Adong. She was one of the fastest runners at our school. During sports competitions, whenever our school competed against others, Adong was always the highlight, and the crowd would cheer for her with excitement. However, as soon as the competitions ended, it seemed no one paid much attention to her. Adong wasn't very strong academically, and in our district, excelling in school and passing exams was seen as the only path to a bright future. Everyone admired Adong's talent and felt proud of her achievements, but at the same time, people pitied her, believing that her future held nothing more than becoming someone's wife in the village and working in the garden. Even Adong herself seemed resigned to this fate.

Then, one day during a sports competition, some judges from the city came to watch the event. They recognized Adong's extraordinary talent and offered her a scholarship to study in America because of her athletic skills. The last we heard of Adong, she was competing internationally as an athlete and doing incredibly well. Adong remains the star of our village and the most successful person to ever come from our community.

Lessons it teaches:
1. **Being in the Right Environment**: Just as a fish thrives and is powerful in water, people are most effective and successful when they are in an environment that supports their growth and strengths. This teaches the importance of seeking out or creating environments that help us flourish.
2. **Recognizing Where You Belong**: The proverb emphasizes the value of understanding where you fit best in life. It suggests that it's crucial to align your actions and efforts with places or situations where your skills and qualities can be fully utilized.
3. **Adapting to Your Surroundings**: It reminds us of the need to adapt to our environment to make the most of our strengths. Being flexible and understanding what's needed in different situations can help us maintain our effectiveness.
4. **Interdependence and Community**: The saying also reflects the importance of being part of a community or network where everyone's unique strengths are recognized and supported. Just as a fish relies on water, people often need a supportive community to truly thrive.

Reflection Questions:

1. How does being in the right environment influence your ability to succeed? Can you think of a time when your environment either helped or hindered your progress?
2. What are some environments or situations where you feel most powerful or effective? How can you create or seek out these spaces more often?
3. Have you ever felt out of place or like a "fish out of water"? How did that experience affect your confidence or performance, and what did you learn from it?
4. What role does your community or support system play in helping you grow and achieve your goals? How can you contribute positively to the strength of that community?
5. How can you adapt when you find yourself in an environment that does not support your strengths? What steps can you take to either improve your surroundings or adjust your approach?

Proverb 12

"Suffering teaches the wisdom of the ancestors."-An African Proverb.

This African proverb emphasizes the idea that enduring hardship can impart deep understanding, wisdom, and lessons that have been passed down from generations before. It suggests that pain and struggles are not meaningless but are opportunities to access a reservoir of ancestral knowledge, resilience, and strength.

A personal Story

Growing up in my small village of Madi Opei, I experienced firsthand the immense hardship brought about by years of violence and unrest. For two decades, my village was ravaged by rebel activity from a group called the Lord's Resistance Army (LRA). They abducted, maimed, raped, killed, and burned down homes. To this day, I still struggle to understand why we had to live in such constant fear for so long.

The rebels planted land mines along the paths to our farms and schools, making everyday tasks perilous. We lived under a strict curfew; by 6 p.m., everyone had to be indoors. Many villagers were forced to live in internally displaced persons (IDP) camps, where they had no means of livelihood and relied entirely on the World Food Program to deliver food every few months. Hunger and starvation were widespread, and the devastation left families broken. Hearing news of death was a daily occurrence, and the air was often filled with the sound of mourning, weeping, and wailing.

Yet, even in the face of such suffering, we found ways to keep our spirits alive. In the evenings, we gathered around the wang oo campfires, singing and dancing to soothe our pain. These gatherings were not only moments of comfort but also times when we learned the wisdom of our ancestors. Through songs and stories, we discovered the strength of resilience, how to make wise decisions in difficult circumstances, and the importance of holding onto hope even in the darkest times.

Lessons it teaches:
1. Resilience: Hardship can build inner strength and resilience, reminding us of the capabilities passed down through generations.
2. Community: Facing difficulties together can forge strong bonds and deepen the understanding of the value of community and shared wisdom.
3. Resourcefulness: Suffering often forces us to be innovative and find solutions that might not have been evident before.
4. Gratitude: Tough times help us appreciate the simple things in life and remember the sacrifices of those who came before us.
5. Perspective: Struggles offer a chance to see the bigger picture, realizing that many before us endured and overcame their challenges.

Reflection Questions:
6. Have you experienced a time when suffering led to personal growth or understanding? How did it change your perspective?
7. What wisdom or lessons have your own ancestors passed down that have helped you navigate hardship?
8. How can we use the challenges we face to strengthen our communities and support one another?
9. In what ways can reflecting on the struggles of previous generations inspire hope and resilience in us today?
10. How do you think modern life either supports or disconnects us from the wisdom of our ancestors? How can we reclaim that connection?

Proverb 13

"Life can be understood backwards but we live it forward."-An African Proverb.

This proverb highlights the idea that we often gain clarity about life events only in hindsight. As we move forward in life, we make decisions and experience situations that might not make sense at the moment. However, looking back, we often see the lessons and reasons behind those experiences. The essence is that while we live in the present and head into an unknown future, the meaning of our journey often only becomes clear when we reflect on the past.

A Personal Story:
Let's go back to the moment when I found myself as a single mother. I remember questioning, "Why me?" Like many young girls, I had dreams of a fairytale wedding: walking down the aisle in a beautiful white dress, marrying the love of my life, and starting a family with three children. But life didn't unfold the way I imagined. The reality was different, and I had to let go of that picture-perfect dream to face the challenges ahead.

Becoming a mother to my daughter gave me a profound sense of purpose. She became the driving force behind everything I did. If not for her, I might never have made it to America, where I was determined to build a better life. I pushed myself harder than I ever thought possible, determined to give her the best future I could. My journey was far from easy, but it taught me resilience and the power of unconditional love. Looking back now, I am incredibly grateful for the life we've built together.

Today, I am using my story to make a difference in my community. By sharing my experiences, I hope to inspire others to find resilience within themselves and hold on to hope, even in the most challenging circumstances. Growing up in my village, where we faced hardships and leaned on each other for strength, shaped who I am today. I carry that sense of community and the lessons of perseverance into everything I do, determined to uplift and empower those around me

Lessons it teaches:
1. **Clarity Comes with Time:** Many life events only make sense when we reflect on them, and that's okay.
2. **Trust the Journey:** Sometimes, things that feel like setbacks are actually guiding us to something better.
3. **Patience and Faith:** We need to have patience and faith in our path, even when the future feels uncertain.
4. **Embrace Uncertainty:** Life will always be full of unknowns, and our growth comes from learning to navigate them.
5. **Reflect and Grow:** Taking time to reflect on past experiences helps us learn and make sense of where we are now.

Reflection Questions:
6. Can you think of a moment in your life that didn't make sense until you looked back on it later? What did you learn from that experience?
7. How do you cope with feelings of uncertainty or disappointment when things don't go as planned?
8. In what ways can reflecting on past experiences help you make better decisions for the future?
9. Why do you think it is hard for us to understand the reasons behind certain life events while we are experiencing them?
10. How can you remind yourself to stay hopeful and open-minded when life feels unpredictable or confusing?

Proverb 14

"Do not hurry the night; the sun will always rise for its own sake."-An African Proverb.

This African proverb speaks to the inevitability of time and natural cycles. It reminds us that everything has its own rhythm and timing. Just as the night cannot rush into dawn, certain aspects of life cannot be forced or rushed. Challenges and dark times will pass, and a new beginning, symbolized by the rising sun, will always come, no matter how difficult the present may seem. Patience and trust in the natural flow of life are key to understanding that what is meant to happen will happen at the right time.

A Personal Story:
There was a time when I found myself in a difficult place, caught between jobs and struggling with serious financial challenges. I had a young child to care for, and the pressure of being a full-time student made things even more complicated. Balancing school and work was exhausting, and I constantly searched for jobs that offered flexible hours to accommodate my academic schedule. Yet, even when I managed to find positions that allowed me to stay in school, the pay was low, and I never seemed to catch up on bills. The constant stress of overdue notices and relentless calls from

service providers only added to my sense of overwhelm.

In those moments, I realized that for both my well-being and my daughter's, I had to make space to be present as a mother. I decided to not let my worries consume every part of me. Each day, after I had exhausted every possible effort to secure work and had completed job applications, I consciously put those troubles aside. It wasn't easy, but I knew I had to disconnect my mind from the stress. Instead of dwelling on what I couldn't control, I waited for my daughter to come home from school, and we would go on little adventures. We'd take walks at the nearby park, try fishing, or capture moments together by taking pictures. Those simple experiences brought us joy and peace, and they reminded me of what truly mattered.

I learned the value of being patient and present. Even though I couldn't hurry time or make the job offers come faster, I could choose how I spent those waiting moments. I had to breathe, to be there for my daughter, and to hold onto hope. Those times taught me resilience and the power of living in the present. It was about finding strength in the in-between spaces and trusting that the process would unfold in its own time.

Lessons Learned:
1. **Patience is Key:** You can't rush certain aspects of life; they will unfold in their own time.
2. **Trust in Natural Cycles:** Just as the sun rises every day, challenges are temporary and will pass.
3. **Personal Growth Takes Time:** Sometimes, the best way to move forward is to take time for self-improvement rather than forcing change.

4. **Trust the Process:** Even in difficult times, have faith that things will improve when the time is right.
5. **Accept Uncertainty:** Life's rhythms are beyond our control, and we must learn to be at peace with the unknown.

Reflection Questions for the Class:

6. Can you think of a time when you tried to rush through a difficult period? What happened, and what did you learn from that experience?
7. In what areas of your life do you find it hardest to be patient, and why do you think that is?
8. How does trusting that things will unfold in their own time change the way you approach challenges?
9. What are some ways you can take care of yourself while waiting for a difficult situation to pass?
10. How do you remind yourself that just as the sun rises every day, your challenges too will eventually pass?

END
Thank you for reading,
I love hearing from my readers, and
I would appreciate if you leave a review for this book.

www.ingramcontent.com/pod-product-compliance
Lightning Source LLC
Chambersburg PA
CBHW071437220526
45469CB00004B/1565